The Super Tasty Keto Vegan Recipe Book

50 Delicious Breakfast and Lunch Recipes for Your Healthy Keto Vegan Diet

Roberta Wells

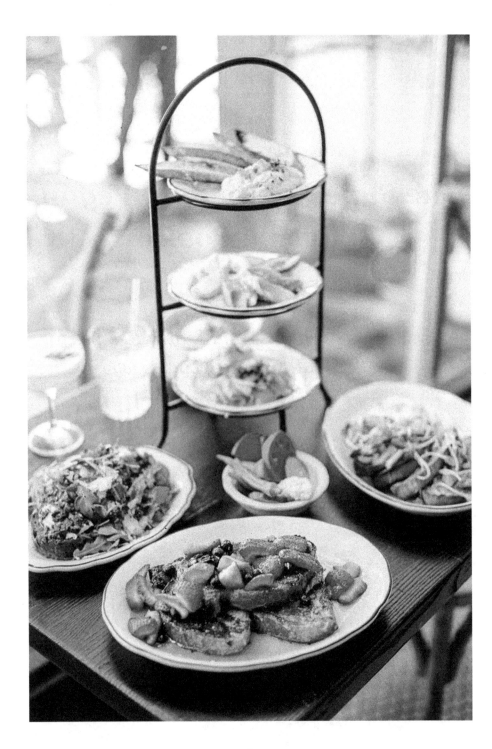

By reading this document, the reader agrees that under no circumstances is the author responsible for any losses, direct or indirect, which are incurred as a result of the use of information contained within this document, including, but not limited to, — errors, omissions, or inaccuracies.

Table of Contents

6

BREAKFAST

Coffee Smoothie

Preparation Time: 5 minutes

Cooking Time: 0 minutes

Servings: 4

Ingredients:

- 4 cups baby spinach
- 4 tablespoons hemp hearts
- 12 Medjool dates, pitted
- 4 tablespoons cashew butter
- 2 cup brewed coffee, chilled
- 6 cups of ice cubes

Directions:

1. Place pitted dates in a medium bowl, cover with hot water and let them soak for 15 minutes.

2. Drain the dates, add them into a food processor along with the remaining ingredients, and then pulse for 1 to 2 minutes until blended, scraping the sides of the container frequently.

3. Distribute the smoothie among glasses and then serve.

Nutrition: 391 Cal 15 g Fat 2 g Saturated Fat 60 g Carbohydrates 6 g Fiber 47 g Sugars 10 g Protein.

Banana Cream Pie and Chia Pudding

Preparation Time: 1 hour and 10 minutes

Cooking Time: 0 minutes

Servings: 4

Ingredients:

- 2 bananas, peeled, mashed
- 2 bananas, peeled, chopped
- 1/2 cup chia seeds
- 2 teaspoons cinnamon
- 4 tablespoons coconut flakes
- 1 cup coconut milk, unsweetened
- 2 tablespoons maple syrup
- 1 cup almond milk, unsweetened

Directions:

1. Take a large bowl, add chia seeds and mashed bananas, add maple syrup and cinnamon, pour in almond and coconut milk and then whisk until well combined.
2. Cover the bowl with lid, and then place it in the refrigerator for a minimum of 1 hour until firm.

3. When ready to eat, distribute pudding evenly among 4 bowls, top with chopped banana, and sprinkle with coconut flakes and then serve.

Nutrition: 350 Cal 17 g Fat 4 g Saturated Fat 37 g Carbohydrates 12 g Fiber 19 g Sugars 5 g Protein.

Brown Rice Breakfast Pudding

Preparation Time: 5 minutes

Cooking Time: 15 minutes

Servings: 4

Ingredients:

- 1 tart apple, cored, chopped
- 1 cup Medjool dates, pitted, chopped
- 3 cups cooked brown rice
- 1/8 teaspoon salt
- ¼ teaspoon ground cloves
- 1 cinnamon stick
- ¼ cup raisins
- ¼ cup slivered almonds, toasted
- 2 cups almond milk, unsweetened

Directions:

1. Take a medium saucepan, place it over medium-low heat, add rice, dates, cloves, and cinnamon, pour in milk, stir until mixed and cook for 12 minutes until thickened.
2. Then remove and discard cinnamon stick, add apple and raisins and then stir in salt.

3. Remove pan from heat, distribute pudding among four bowls and top with almonds.

4. Serve straight away.

Nutrition: 391 Cal 4.8 g Fat 0.6 g Saturated Fat 81.1 g Carbohydrates 5.7 g Fiber 24.8 g Sugars 6 g Protein.

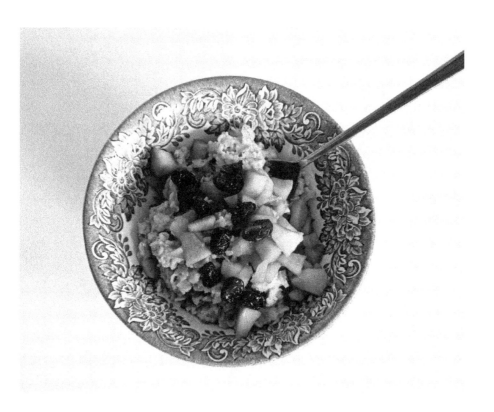

Carrot Cake Oats

Preparation Time: 6 hours and 10 minutes

Cooking Time: 0 minutes

Servings: 4

Ingredients:

- ¼ cup shredded carrot
- 1/3 cup rolled oats
- 2 tablespoons chopped pineapple
- 1 tablespoon shredded coconut, unsweetened and more for topping
- 1 tablespoon ground flaxseed
- 1 tablespoon raisins and more for topping
- 2 tablespoons maple syrup and more for topping
- 1/8 teaspoon ground nutmeg
- ¼ teaspoon ground cinnamon and more for topping
- ¼ teaspoon vanilla extract, unsweetened
- 1 tablespoon chopped walnuts and more for topping
- ½ cup almond milk, unsweetened

Directions:

1. Take a large bowl, place all the ingredients in it, and stir until well mixed.
2. Cover the bowl with lid, and then place it in the refrigerator for a minimum of a minimum of 6 hours.
3. When ready to eat, distribute oats mixture evenly among 4 bowls, top with some shredded coconut, raisins, and walnuts, sprinkle with cinnamon, drizzle with maple syrup and then serve.

Nutrition: 242 Cal 9 g Fat 2 g Saturated Fat 35 g Carbohydrates 6 g Fiber 12 g Sugars 7 g Protein.

Chocolate Chip and Coconut Pancakes

Preparation Time: 10 minutes

Cooking Time: 40 minutes

Servings: 8

Ingredients:

- 1¼ cups buckwheat flour
- 1 tablespoon flaxseeds
- 2 tablespoons coconut flakes, unsweetened
- ¼ cup rolled oats
- 1/8 teaspoon sea salt
- 1 tablespoon baking powder
- 1/3 cup mini chocolate chips, vegan
- ¼ cup maple syrup
- 1 teaspoon vanilla extract, unsweetened
- ½ cup applesauce, unsweetened
- 1 cup almond milk, unsweetened
- ½ cup of water
- 2 bananas, peeled, sliced

Directions:

1. Take a small saucepan, place it over medium heat, add flaxseeds, pour in water, and then

cook for 4 to 5 minutes until sticky mixture comes together.

2. Strain the flaxseeds mixture immediately into a cup, discard the seeds, and set aside the collected flax water until required.

3. Take a large bowl, add buckwheat flour and oats in it, and then stir in salt, baking powder, and coconut until mixed.

4. Take a medium bowl, add 2 tablespoons of reserved flax water along with maple syrup and vanilla, pour in applesauce and milk, and whisk until combined.

5. Pour the milk mixture into the flour mixture, whisk well until thick batter comes together, and then fold in chocolate chips.

6. Take a griddle pan, place it over medium-low heat, spray it with oil and when hot, pour in 1/3 cup of the prepared batter, spread it gently and cook for 5 to 7 minutes until the bottom turns golden brown; pour in more batter if there is a space on the pan.

7. Flip the pancake, continue cooking for 5 minutes, and when done, transfer pancake to a plate and then repeat with the remaining batter.

8. Serve pancakes with sliced bananas.

Nutrition: 190 Cal 14 g Fat 6 g Saturated Fat 8 g Carbohydrates 2 g Fiber 4 g Sugars 8 g Protein.

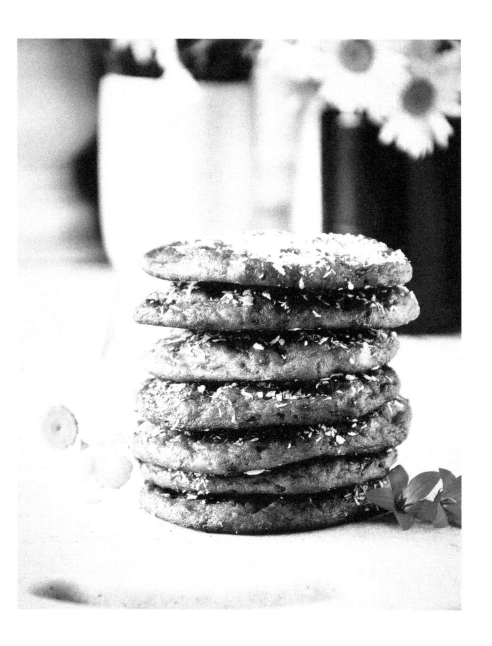

Berries and Banana Smoothie Bowl

Preparation Time: 5 minutes

Cooking Time: 0 minutes

Servings: 4

Ingredients:

For the Smoothie:

- 4 cups frozen mixed berries
- 4 small frozen banana, sliced
- 4 scoops of vanilla protein powder
- 12 tablespoons almond milk, unsweetened

For the Toppings:

- 4 tablespoons chia seeds
- 4 tablespoons shredded coconut, unsweetened
- 4 tablespoons hemp seeds
- ½ cup Granola
- Fresh strawberries, sliced, as needed

Directions:

1. Add mixed berries into a food processor along with banana and then pulse at low speed for 1 to 2 minutes until broken.
2. Add remaining ingredients for the smoothie and then pulse again for 1 minute at low speed

until creamy, scraping the sides of the container frequently.

3. Distribute the smoothie among four bowls, then top with chia seeds, coconut, hemp seeds, granola, and strawberries and serve.

Nutrition: 214 Cal 2.5 g Fat 1.6 g Saturated Fat 47.5 g Carbohydrates 8.8 g Fiber 26 g Sugars 2.8 g Protein.

Mint Chocolate Protein Smoothie

Preparation Time: 5 minutes

Cooking Time: 0 minutes

Servings: 4

Ingredients:

- 4 tablespoons ground flaxseed
- 4 cups fresh spinach
- 4 frozen banana, sliced
- 4 scoops of chocolate protein powder
- 4 tablespoons chopped dark chocolate, vegan
- ½ cup melted dark chocolate
- 1 teaspoon peppermint extract, unsweetened
- 4 tablespoons honey
- 3 cups almond milk, unsweetened
- 1 cup ice cubed

Directions:

1. Add all the ingredients in the order into a food processor or blender and then pulse for 1 to 2 minutes until blended, scraping the sides of the container frequently.
2. Distribute the smoothie among glasses and then serve.

Nutrition: 480.5 Cal 20.3 g Fat 8.4 g Saturated Fat 45.6 g Carbohydrates 9.7 g Fiber 22.5 g Sugars 31.2 g Protein;

Sunrise Smoothie

Preparation Time: 5 minutes

Cooking Time: 0 minutes

Servings: 4

Ingredients:

- 4 tablespoons chia seed
- 2 frozen banana
- 2 lemon, peeled
- 2 cups diced carrots
- 4 clementine, peeled
- 4 cups frozen strawberries, unsweetened
- 12 tablespoons pomegranate tendrils
- 2 cup almond milk, unsweetened

Directions:

1. Add all the ingredients in the order into a food processor or blender and then pulse for 1 to 2 minutes until blended, scraping the sides of the container frequently.
2. Distribute the smoothie among glasses and then serve.

Nutrition: 274 Cal 5.4 g Fat 0.5 g Saturated Fat 57.3 g Carbohydrates 13.3 g Fiber 33.8 g Sugars 0.5 g Protein.

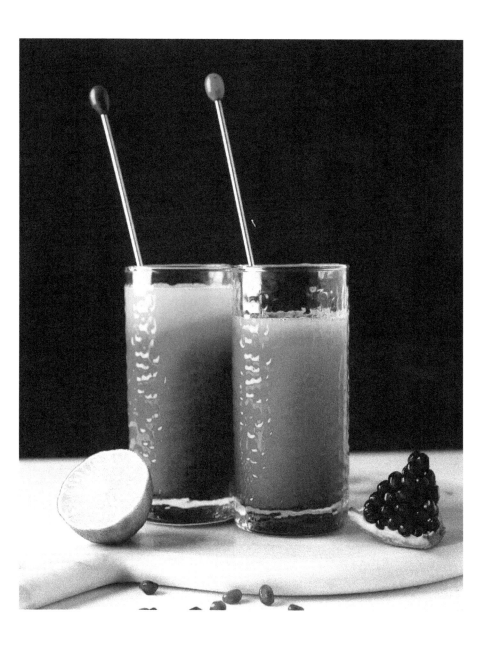

Sunshine Orange Smoothie

Preparation Time: 5 minutes

Cooking Time: 0 minutes

Servings: 4

Ingredients:

- 2 medium oranges, zested, juiced
- 4 frozen bananas
- 4 tablespoons goji berries
- ½ cup hemp seeds
- 1 teaspoon grated ginger
- 1 cup almond milk, unsweetened
- ½ cup of ice cubes

Directions:

1. Add all the ingredients in the order into a food processor or blender and then pulse for 1 to 2 minutes until blended, scraping the sides of the container frequently.
2. Distribute the smoothie among glasses and then serve.

Nutrition: 131 Cal 2.3 g Fat 0.3 g Saturated Fat 26.7 g Carbohydrates 4.4 g Fiber 11 g Sugars 2.6 g Protein.

Chocolate and Hazelnut Smoothie

Preparation Time: 5 minutes

Cooking Time: 0 minutes

Servings: 4

Ingredients:

- 1 frozen banana
- 1 cup hazelnuts, unsalted, roasted
- 8 teaspoons maple syrup
- 4 tablespoons cocoa powder, unsweetened
- 1/2 teaspoon hazelnut extract, unsweetened
- 2 cups almond milk, unsweetened
- 1 cup of ice cubes

Directions:

1. Add all the ingredients in the order into a food processor or blender and then pulse for 1 to 2 minutes until blended, scraping the sides of the container frequently.
2. Distribute the smoothie among glasses and then serve.

Nutrition: 198 Cal 12 g Fat 1 g Saturated Fat 21 g Carbohydrates 5 g Fiber 12 g Sugars 5 g Protein.

Blueberry Oatmeal Smoothie

Preparation Time: 5 minutes

Cooking Time: 0 minutes

Servings: 4

Ingredients:

- 2 cups frozen blueberries
- 1 cup old-fashioned oats
- 2 teaspoons cinnamon
- 2 tablespoons maple syrup
- 1 cup spinach
- 2 cup almond milk, unsweetened
- 8 ice cubes

Directions:

1. Add all the ingredients in the order into a food processor or blender and then pulse for 1 to 2 minutes until blended, scraping the sides of the container frequently.
2. Distribute the smoothie among glasses and then serve.

Nutrition: 194 Cal 5 g Fat 3 g Saturated Fat 34 g Carbohydrates 5 g Fiber 15 g Sugars 5 g Protein.

Orange French Toast

Preparation Time: 5 minutes

Cooking Time: 30 minutes

Servings: 8 servings

Ingredients:

- 2 cups of plant milk (unflavored)
- Four tablespoon maple syrup
- 11/2 tablespoon cinnamon
- Salt (optional)
- 1 cup flour (almond)
- 1 tablespoon orange zest
- 8 bread slices

Directions:

1. Turn the oven and heat to 400-degree F afterwards.
2. In a cup, add ingredients: and whisk until the batter is smooth.
3. Dip each piece of bread into the paste and permit to soak for a couple of seconds.
4. Put in the pan, and cook until lightly browned.

5. Put the toast on the cookie sheet and bake for ten to fifteen minutes in the oven, until it is crispy.

Nutrition: Calories: 129 Fat: 1.1g Carbohydrates: 21.5g Protein: 7.9g

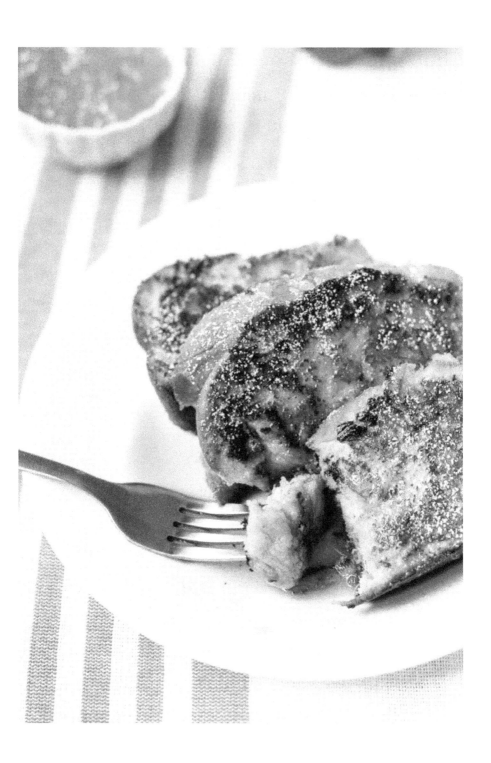

Chocolate Chip Coconut Pancakes

Preparation Time: 5 minutes

Cooking Time: 30 minutes

Servings: 8 servings

Ingredients:

- 11/4 cup oats
- 2 teaspoons coconut flakes
- 2 cup plant milk
- 11/4 cup maple syrup
- 11/3 cup of chocolate chips
- 2 1/4 cups buckwheat flour
- 2 teaspoon baking powder
- 1 teaspoon vanilla essence
- 2 teaspoon flaxseed meal
- Salt (optional)

Directions:

1. Put the flaxseed and cook over medium heat until the paste becomes a little moist.
2. Remove seeds.
3. Stir the buckwheat, oats, coconut chips, baking powder and salt with each other in a wide dish.

4. In a large dish, stir together the retained flax water with the sugar, maple syrup, vanilla essence.

5. Transfer the wet mixture to the dry and shake to combine

6. Place over medium heat the nonstick grill pan.

7. Pour 1/4 cup flour onto the grill pan with each pancake, and scatter gently.

8. Cook for five to six minutes, before the pancakes appear somewhat crispy.

Nutrition: Calories: 198 Fat: 9.1g Carbohydrates: 11.5g Protein: 7.9g

Apple-Lemon Bowl

Preparation Time: 5 minutes

Cooking Time: 15 minutes

Servings: 1-2 servings

Ingredients:

- 6 apples
- 3 tablespoons walnuts
- 7 dates
- Lemon juice
- 1/2 teaspoon cinnamon

Directions:

1. Root the apples, then break them into wide bits.
2. In a food cup, put seeds, part of the lime juice, almonds, spices and three-quarters of the apples. Thinly slice until finely ground.
3. Apply the remaining apples and lemon juice and make slices.

Nutrition: Calories: 249 Fat: 5.1g Carbohydrates: 71.5g Protein: 7.9g

Breakfast Scramble

Preparation Time: 10 minutes

Cooking Time: 30 minutes

Servings: 6 servings

Ingredients:

- 1 red onion1 to
- 2 tablespoons soy sauce
- 2 cups sliced mushrooms
- Salt to taste
- 11/2 teaspoon black pepper
- 11/2 teaspoons turmeric
- 1/4 teaspoon cayenne
- 3 cloves garlic
- 1 red bell pepper
- 1 large head cauliflower
- 1 green bell pepper

Directions:

1. In a small pan, put all vegetables and cook until crispy.
2. Stir in the cauliflower and cook for four to six minutes or until it smooth.

3. Add spices to the pan and cook for another five minutes.

Nutrition: Calories: 199 Fat: 1.1g Carbohydrates: 14.5g Protein: 7.9g

Black Bean and Sweet Potato Hash

Preparation Time: 10 minutes

Cooking Time: 30 minutes

Servings: 4 servings

Ingredients:

- 1 cup onion (chopped)
- 1/3 Cup vegetable broth
- 2 garlic (minced)
- 1 cup cooked black beans
- 2 teaspoons hot chili powder
- 2 cups chopped sweet potatoes

Directions:

1. Put the onions in a saucepan over medium heat and add the seasoning and mix.
2. Add potatoes and chili flakes, then mix.
3. Cook for around 12 minutes more until the vegetables are cooked thoroughly.
4. Add the green onion, beans, and salt
5. Cook for more 2 minutes and serve.

Nutrition: Calories: 239 Fat: 1.1g Carbohydrates: 71.5g Protein: 7.9g

Chocolate Peanut Butter Shake

Preparation Time: 5 minutes

Cooking Time: 5 minutes

Servings: 2 servings

Ingredients:

- 2 bananas
- 3 Tablespoons peanut butter
- 1 cup almond milk
- 3 Tablespoons cacao powder

Directions:

1. Combine in a blender until smooth.

Nutrition: Calories: 149 Fat: 1.1g Carbohydrates: 1.5g Protein: 7.9g

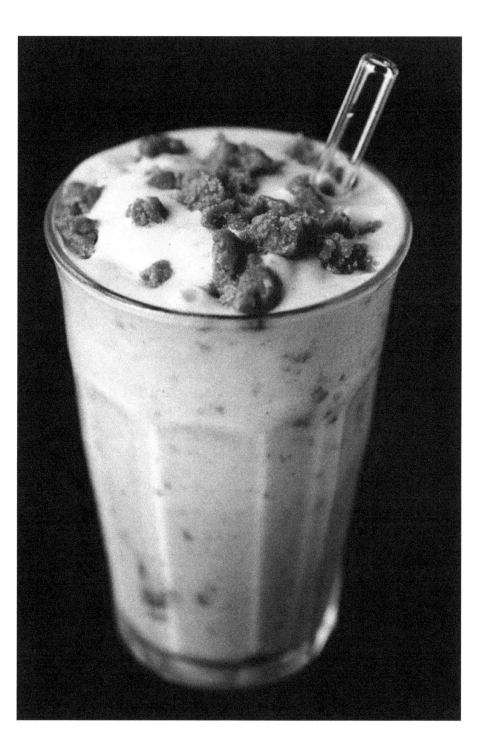

Breakfast Cookies

Preparation Time: 10 minutes

Cooking Time: 6 minutes

Servings: 24-32

Ingredients:

Dry **Ingredients**:

- ½ teaspoon baking powder
- 2 cups rolled oats
- ½ teaspoon baking soda

Wet **Ingredients:**

- 1 teaspoon pure vanilla extract
- 2 flax eggs (2 tablespoons ground flaxseed and around 6 tablespoons of water, mix and put aside for 15 minutes)
- 2 tablespoons melted coconut oil
- 2 tablespoons pure maple syrup
- ½ cup natural creamy peanut butter
- 2 ripe bananas

Add-in **Ingredients:**

- ½ cup finely chopped walnuts
- ½ cup raisins

Optional Topping:

- 2 tablespoons chopped walnuts
- 2 tablespoons raisins

Directions:

1. Preheat the oven to 325 degrees F, and then use parchment paper to line a baking sheet and put aside.

2. Add the bananas in a large bowl, and then use a fork to mash them until smooth. Add in the other wet ingredients and mix until well incorporated.

3. Add the dry ingredients and then use a rubber spatula to stir and fold them into the dry ingredients until well mixed. Stir in the walnuts and raisins.

4. Scoop the cookie dough onto the prepared baking sheet making sure that you leave adequate space between the cookies.

5. Bake in the preheated oven for around 12 minutes. Once ready, let the cookies cool on the baking sheet for around 10 minutes.

6. Lift the cookies carefully from the baking sheet onto a cooling rack to further cool.

7. Store the cookies in an airtight container in the fridge or at room temperature for up to one week.

Nutrition: Calories 565 Fat 6 Carbs 32 Protein 8

Vegan Breakfast Biscuits

Preparation Time: 10 minutes

Cooking Time: 10 min

Servings: 6

Ingredients:

- cups Almond Flour - quantity not mentioned
- 1 tbsp. Baking Powder
- ¼ teaspoon Salt
- ½ teaspoon Onion Powder
- ½ cup Coconut Milk
- ¼ cup Nutritional Yeast
- 2 tbsp. Ground Flax Seeds
- ¼ cup Olive Oil

Directions:

1. Preheat oven to 450F.
2. Whisk together all ingredients in a bowl.
3. Divide the batter into a pre-greased muffin tin.
4. Bake for 10 minutes.

Nutrition: Calories 432 Fat 5 Carbs 13 Protein 8

LUNCH

Rainbow Taco Boats

Preparation Time: 10 minutes

Cooking Time: 0 minutes

Servings: 4

Ingredients:

- 1 head romaine lettuce, destemmed

For the Filling:

- 1/2 cup alfalfa sprouts
- 1 medium avocado, peeled, pitted, cubed
- 1 cup shredded carrots
- 1 cup halved cherry tomatoes
- 3/4 cup sliced red cabbage
- 1/2 cup sprouted hummus dip
- 1 tablespoon hemp seeds

For the Sauce:

- 1 tablespoon maple syrup
- 1/3 cup tahini
- 1/8 teaspoon sea salt
- 2 tablespoons lemon juice
- 3 tablespoons water

Directions:

1. Prepare the sauce and for this, take a medium bowl, add all the ingredients in it and whisk until well combined.

2. Assemble the boats and for this, arrange lettuce leaves in twelve portions, top each with hummus, and the remaining ingredients for the filling.

3. Serve with prepared sauce.

Nutrition: 314 Cal 23.6 g Fat 4 g Saturated Fat 23.2 g Carbohydrates 9.3 g Fiber 6.2 g Sugars 8 g Protein.

Eggplant Sandwich

Preparation Time: 10 minutes

Cooking Time: 25 minutes

Servings: 4

Ingredients:

For the Sandwich:

- 2 ciabatta buns
- 1 medium eggplant, peeled, sliced, soaked in salted water
- 1 medium tomato, sliced
- 1/2 of a medium cucumber, sliced
- 1/2 cup arugula
- 4 tablespoons mayo

For the Marinade:

- 1 teaspoon agave syrup
- 1/4 teaspoon salt
- 1/4 teaspoon ground black pepper
- 1 teaspoon smoked paprika
- 1 tablespoon soy sauce
- 1 tablespoon olive oil

Directions:

1. Switch on the oven, then set it to 350 degrees F and let it preheat.

2. Prepare the marinade and for this, take a small bowl, place all the ingredients in it and whisk until combined.

3. Drain the eggplant slices, pat dry with a kitchen towel, and brush with prepared marinade, arrange them on a baking sheet and then bake for 20 minutes until done.

4. Assemble the sandwich and for this, slice the bread in half lengthwise, then spread mayonnaise in the bottom half of the bun and top with baked eggplant slices, tomato, and cucumber slices, and sprinkle with salt and black pepper.

5. Top with arugula leaves, cover with the top half of the bun, and then cover with aluminum foil.

6. Preheat the grill over medium-high heat setting and when hot, place prepared

sandwiches and grill for 3 to 5 minutes until toasted.

7. Cut each sandwich through the foil into half and serve.

Nutrition: 688 Cal 15 g Fat 2 g Saturated Fat 118 g Carbohydrates 7 g Fiber 7 g Sugars 21 g Protein.

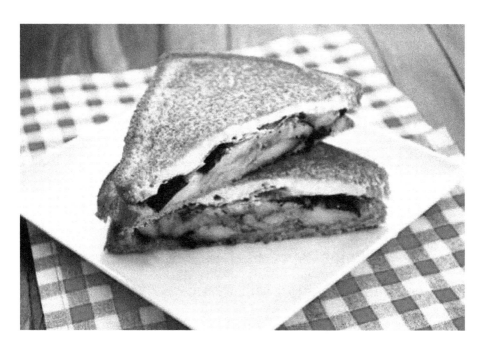

Lentil, Cauliflower and Grape Salad

Preparation Time: 10 minutes

Cooking Time: 25 minutes

Servings: 4

Ingredients:

- For the Cauliflower:
- 1 medium head of cauliflower, cut into florets
- 1/4 teaspoon sea salt
- 1 1/2 tablespoons curry powder
- 1 1/2 tablespoons melted coconut oil

For the Tahini Dressing:

- 2 tablespoons tahini
- 1/8 teaspoon salt
- 1.8 teaspoon ground black pepper
- 4 1/2 tablespoons green curry paste
- 1 tablespoon maple syrup
- 2 tablespoons lemon juice
- 2 tablespoons water

For the Salad:

- 1 cup cooked lentils
- 4 tablespoons chopped cilantro
- 1 cup red grapes, halved

- 6 cups mixed greens

Directions:

1. Switch on the oven, then set it to 400 degrees F and let it preheat.

2. Prepare the cauliflower and for this, take a medium bowl, place cauliflower florets in it, drizzle with oil, season with salt and curry powder, toss until mixed.

3. Take a baking sheet, line it with parchment sheet, spread cauliflower florets in it, and then bake for 25 minutes until tender and nicely golden brown.

4. Meanwhile, prepare the tahini dressing and for this, take a medium bowl, place all its ingredients and whisk until combined, set aside until required.

5. Assemble the salad and for this, take a large salad bowl, add roasted cauliflower florets, lentils, grapes, and mixed greens, drizzle with prepared tahini dressing and toss until well combined.

6. Serve straight away.

Nutrition: 420 Cal 14 g Fat 5 g Saturated Fat 37.6 g Carbohydrates 9.8 g Fiber 12.8 g Sugars 10.8 g Protein.

Loaded Kale Salad

Preparation Time: 10 minutes

Cooking Time: 30 minutes

Servings: 4

Ingredients:

- 1 ½ cup cooked quinoa

For The Vegetables:

- 1 whole beet, peeled, sliced
- 4 large carrots, peeled, chopped
- 1/2 teaspoon curry powder
- 1/8 teaspoon sea salt
- 2 tablespoons melted coconut oil

For The Dressing:

- ¼ teaspoon of sea salt
- 2 tablespoons maple syrup
- 3 tablespoons lemon juice
- 1/3 cup tahini
- 1/4 cup water

For the Salad:

- 1/2 cup sprouts
- 1 medium avocado, peeled, pitted, cubed
- 1/2 cup chopped cherry tomatoes

- 8 cups chopped kale
- 1/4 cup hemp seeds

Directions:

1. Switch on the oven, then set it to 375 degrees F and let it preheat.
2. Take a baking sheet, place beets and carrots on it, drizzle with oil, season with curry powder and salt, toss until coated, and then bake for 30 minutes until tender and golden brown.
3. Meanwhile, prepare the dressing and for this, take a small bowl, place all the ingredients in it and whisk until well combined, set aside until required.
4. Assemble the salad and for this, take a large salad bowl, place kale leaves in it, add remaining ingredients for the salad along with roasted vegetables, drizzle with prepared dressing and toss until combined.
5. Serve straight away.

Nutrition: 472 Cal 22.8 g Fat 3.8 g Saturated Fat 58.7 g Carbohydrates 12.5 g Fiber 9.2 g Sugars 14.6 g Protein.

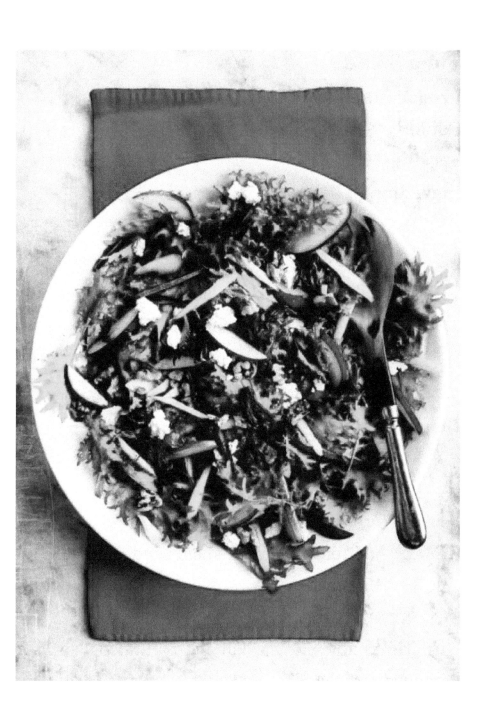

Tuna Salad

Preparation Time: 10 minutes

Cooking Time: 0 minutes

Servings: 4

Ingredients:

- 1/2 cup chopped celery
- 3 cups cooked chickpeas
- 1 tablespoon capers, chopped
- 2 tablespoons sweet pickle relish
- 1 tablespoon yellow mustard paste
- 2 tablespoons mayonnaise

Directions:

1. Take a medium bowl, place chickpeas in it, add mustard and mayonnaise and mash by using a fork until peas are broken.
2. Add remaining ingredients and stir until well combined.
3. Serve straight away.

Nutrition: 207 Cal 7 g Fat 1 g Saturated Fat 27 g Carbohydrates 8 g Fiber 1 g Sugars 9 g Protein.

White Bean and Artichoke Sandwich

Preparation Time: 15 minutes

Cooking Time: 10 minutes

Servings: 4

Ingredients:

- 1 ¼ cooked white beans
- ½ cup cashew nuts
- 6 artichoke hearts, chopped
- ¼ cup sunflower seeds, hulled
- 1 clove of garlic, peeled
- ¼ teaspoon salt
- ¼ teaspoon ground black pepper
- 1 teaspoon dried rosemary
- 1 lemon, grated
- 6 tablespoons almond milk, unsweetened
- 8 pieces of rustic bread

Directions:

1. Soak cashew nuts in warm water for 10 minutes, then drain them and transfer into a food processor.

2. Add garlic, salt, black pepper, rosemary, lemon zest, and milk and then pulse for 2

minutes until smooth, scraping the sides of the container frequently.

3. Take a medium bowl, place beans in it, mash them by using a fork, then add sunflower seeds and artichokes and stir until mixed.

4. Pour in cashew nuts dressing, stir until coated, and taste to adjust seasoning.

5. Take a medium skillet pan, place it over medium heat, add bread slices, and cook for 3 minutes per side until toasted.

6. Spread white beans mixture on one side of four bread slices and then cover with the other four slices.

7. Serve straight away.

Nutrition: 220 Cal 8 g Fat 1 g Saturated Fat 28 g Carbohydrates 8 g Fiber 2 g Sugars 12 g Protein.

Crusty Grilled Corn

Preparation Time: 10 minutes

Cooking Time: 15 minutes

Servings: 4

Ingredients:

- 2 corn cobs
- 1/3 cup Vegenaise
- 1 small handful cilantro
- ½ cup breadcrumbs
- 1 teaspoon lemon juice

Directions:

1. Preheat the gas grill on high heat.
2. Add corn grill to the grill and continue grilling until it turns golden-brown on all sides.
3. Mix the Vegenaise, cilantro, breadcrumbs, and lemon juice in a bowl.
4. Add grilled corn cobs to the crumbs mixture.
5. Toss well then serve.

Nutrition: Calories: 253 Total Fat: 13g Protein: 31g Total Carbs: 3g Fiber: 0g Net Carbs: 3g

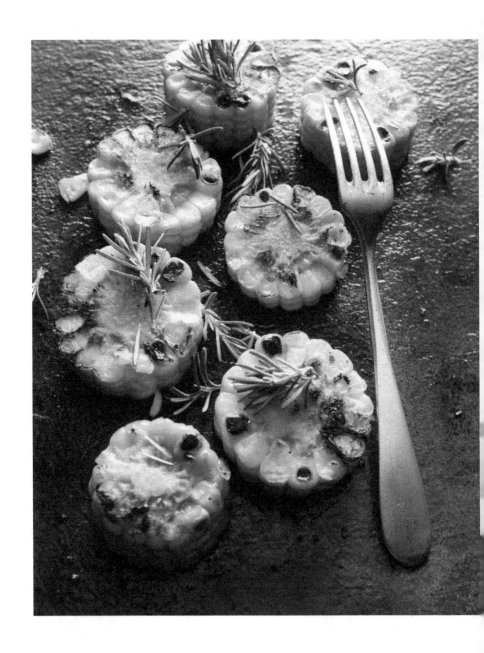

Grilled Carrots with Chickpea Salad

Preparation Time: 10 minutes

Cooking Time: 10 minutes

Servings: 8

Ingredients:

- Carrots
- 8 large carrots
- 1 tablespoon oil
- 1 ½ teaspoon salt
- 1 teaspoon dried oregano
- 1 teaspoon dried thyme
- 2 teaspoon paprika powder
- 1 ½ tablespoon soy sauce
- ½ cup of water
- Chickpea Salad
- 14 oz. canned chickpeas
- 3 medium pickles
- 1 small onion
- A big handful of lettuce
- 1 teaspoon apple cider vinegar
- ½ teaspoon dried oregano

- ½ teaspoon salt
- Ground black pepper, to taste
- ½ cup vegan cream

Directions:

1. Toss the carrots with all its ingredients in a bowl.
2. Thread one carrot on a stick and place it on a plate.
3. Preheat the grill over high heat.
4. Grill the carrots for 2 minutes per side on the grill.
5. Toss the ingredients for the salad in a large salad bowl.
6. Slice grilled carrots and add them on top of the salad.
7. Serve fresh.

Nutrition: Calories: 661 Total Fat: 68g Carbs: 17g Net Carbs: 7g Fiber: 2g Protein: 4g

Grilled Avocado Guacamole

Preparation Time: 10 minutes

Cooking Time: 20 minutes

Servings: 4

Ingredients:

- ½ teaspoon olive oil
- 1 lime, halved
- ½ onion, halved
- 1 serrano chile, halved, stemmed, and seeded
- 3 Haas avocados, skin on
- 2–3 tablespoons fresh cilantro, chopped
- ½ teaspoon smoked salt

Directions:

1. Preheat the grill over medium heat.
2. Brush the grilling grates with olive oil and place chile, onion, and lime on it.
3. Grill the onion for 10 minutes, chile for 5 minutes, and lime for 2 minutes.
4. Transfer the veggies to a large bowl.
5. Now cut the avocados in half and grill them for 5 minutes.
6. Mash the flesh of the grilled avocado in a bowl.

7. Chop the other grilled veggies and add them to the avocado mash.

8. Stir in remaining ingredients and mix well.

9. Serve.

Nutrition: Calories: 165 Total Fat: 17g Carbs: 4g Net Carbs: 2g Fiber: 1g Protein: 1g

Tofu Hoagie Rolls

Preparation Time: 10 minutes

Cooking Time: 20 minutes

Servings: 6

Ingredients:

- ½ cup vegetable broth
- ¼ cup hot sauce
- 1 tablespoon vegan butter
- 1 (16 ounce) package tofu, pressed and diced
- 4 cups cabbage, shredded
- 2 medium apples, grated
- 1 medium shallot, grated
- 6 tablespoons vegan mayonnaise
- 1 tablespoon apple cider vinegar
- Salt and black pepper
- 4 6-inch hoagie rolls, toasted

Directions:

1. In a saucepan, combine broth with butter and hot sauce and bring to a boil.
2. Add tofu and reduce the heat to a simmer.
3. Cook for 10 minutes then remove from heat and let sit for 10 minutes to marinate.

4. Toss cabbage and rest of the ingredients in a salad bowl.

5. Prepare and set up a grill on medium heat.

6. Drain the tofu and grill for 5 minutes per side.

7. Lay out the toasted hoagie rolls and add grilled tofu to each hoagie

8. Add the cabbage mixture evenly between them then close it.

9. Serve.

Nutrition: Calories: 111 Total Fat: 11g Carbs: 5g Net Carbs: 1g Fiber: 0g Protein: 1g

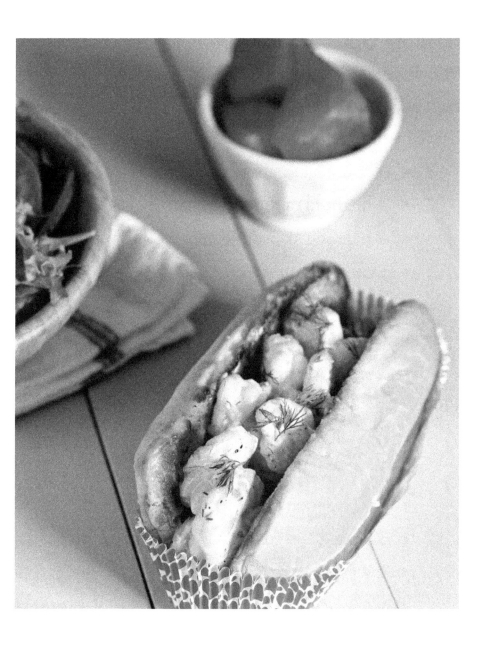

Grilled Seitan with Creole Sauce

Preparation Time: 10 minutes

Cooking Time: 14 minutes

Servings: 4

Ingredients:

Grilled Seitan Kebabs:

- 4 cups seitan, diced
- 2 medium onions, diced into squares
- 8 bamboo skewers
- 1 can coconut milk
- 2½ tablespoons creole spice
- 2 tablespoons tomato paste
- 2 cloves of garlic

Creole Spice Mix:

- 2 tablespoons paprika
- 12 dried peri chili peppers
- 1 tablespoon salt
- 1 tablespoon freshly ground pepper
- 2 teaspoons dried thyme
- 2 teaspoons dried oregano

Directions:

1. Prepare the creole seasoning by blending all its ingredients and preserve in a sealable jar.
2. Thread seitan and onion on the bamboo skewers in an alternating pattern.
3. On a baking sheet, mix coconut milk with creole seasoning, tomato paste and garlic.
4. Soak the skewers in the milk marinade for 2 hours.
5. Prepare and set up a grill over medium heat.
6. Grill the skewers for 7 minutes per side.
7. Serve.

Nutrition: Calories: 407 Total Fat: 42g Carbs: 13g Net Carbs: 6g Fiber: 1g Protein: 4g

Mushroom Steaks

Preparation Time: 10 minutes

Cooking Time: 24 minutes

Servings: 4

Ingredients:

- 1 tablespoon vegan butter
- ½ cup vegetable broth
- ½ small yellow onion, diced
- 1 large garlic clove, minced
- 3 tablespoons balsamic vinegar
- 1 tablespoon mirin
- ½ tablespoon soy sauce
- ½ tablespoon tomato paste
- 1 teaspoon dried thyme
- ½ teaspoon dried basil
- A dash of ground black pepper
- 2 large, whole portobello mushrooms

Directions:

1. Melt butter in a saucepan over medium heat and stir in half of the broth.
2. Bring to a simmer then add garlic and onion. Cook for 8 minutes.

3. Whisk the rest of the ingredients except the mushrooms in a bowl.

4. Add this mixture to the onion in the pan and mix well.

5. Bring this filling to a simmer then remove from the heat.

6. Clean the mushroom caps inside and out and divide the filling between the mushrooms.

7. Place the mushrooms on a baking sheet and top them with remaining sauce and broth.

8. Cover with foil then place it on a grill to smoke.

9. Cover the grill and broil for 16 minutes over indirect heat.

10. Serve warm.

Nutrition: Calories: 887 Total Fat: 93g Carbs: 29g Net Carbs: 13g Fiber: 4g Protein: 8g

Grilled Portobello

Preparation Time: 10 minutes

Cooking Time: 8 minutes

Servings: 04

Ingredients:

- 4 portobello mushrooms
- ¼ cup soy sauce
- ¼ cup tomato sauce
- 2 tablespoons maple syrup
- 1 tablespoon molasses
- 2 tablespoons minced garlic
- 1 tablespoon onion powder
- 1 pinch salt and pepper

Directions:

1. Mix all the ingredients except mushrooms in a bowl.
2. Add mushrooms to this marinade and mix well to coat.
3. Cover and marinate for 1 hour.
4. Prepare and set up the grill at medium heat. Grease it with cooking spray.
5. Grill the mushroom for 4 minutes per side.

6. Serve

Nutrition: Calories: 404 Total Fat: 43g Carbs: 8g Net
Carbs: 4g Fiber: 1g Protein: 4g

Wok Fried Broccoli

Preparation Time: 10 minutes

Cooking Time: 16 minutes

Servings: 02

Ingredients:

- 3 ounces whole, blanched peanuts
- 2 tablespoons olive oil
- 1 banana shallot, sliced
- 10 ounces broccoli, trimmed and cut into florets
- ¼ red pepper, julienned
- ½ yellow pepper, julienned
- 1 teaspoon soy sauce

Directions:

1. Toast peanuts on a baking sheet for 15 minutes at 350 degrees F.
2. In a wok, add oil and shallots and sauté for 10 minutes.
3. Toss in broccoli and peppers.
4. Stir fry for 3 minutes then add the rest of the ingredients.
5. Cook for 3 additional minutes and serve.

Nutrition: Calories: 391 Total Fat: 39g Carbs: 15g Net Carbs: 5g Fiber: 2g Protein: 6g

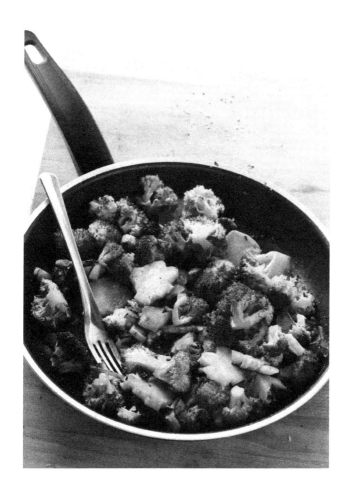

Broccoli & Brown Rice Satay

Preparation Time: 10 minutes

Cooking Time: 10 minutes

Servings: 4

Ingredients:

- 6 trimmed broccoli florets, halved
- 1-inch piece of ginger, shredded
- 2 garlic cloves, shredded
- 1 red onion, sliced
- 1 roasted red pepper, cut into cubes
- 2 teaspoons olive oil
- 1 teaspoon mild chili powder
- 1 tablespoon reduced salt soy sauce
- 1 tablespoon maple syrup
- 1 cup cooked brown rice

Directions:

1. Boil broccoli in water for 4 minutes then drain immediately.
2. In a pan add olive oil, ginger, onion, and garlic.
3. Stir fry for 2 minutes then add the rest of the ingredients.
4. Cook for 3 minutes then serve.

Nutrition: Calories: 196 Total Fat: 20g Carbs: 8g Net Carbs: 3g Fiber: 1g Protein: 3g

Sautéed Sesame Spinach

Preparation Time: 1 hr. 10 minutes

Cooking Time: 3 minutes

Servings: 04

Ingredients:

- 1 tablespoon toasted sesame oil
- ½ tablespoon soy sauce
- ½ teaspoon toasted sesame seeds, crushed
- ½ teaspoon rice vinegar
- ½ teaspoon golden caster sugar
- 1 garlic clove, grated
- 8 ounces spinach, stem ends trimmed

Directions:

1. Sauté spinach in a pan until it is wilted.
2. Whisk the sesame oil, garlic, sugar, vinegar, sesame seeds, soy sauce and black pepper together in a bowl.
3. Stir in spinach and mix well.
4. Cover and refrigerate for 1 hour.
5. Serve.

Nutrition: Calories: 677 Total Fat: 60g Carbs: 71g Net Carbs: 7g Fiber: 0g; Protein: 20g

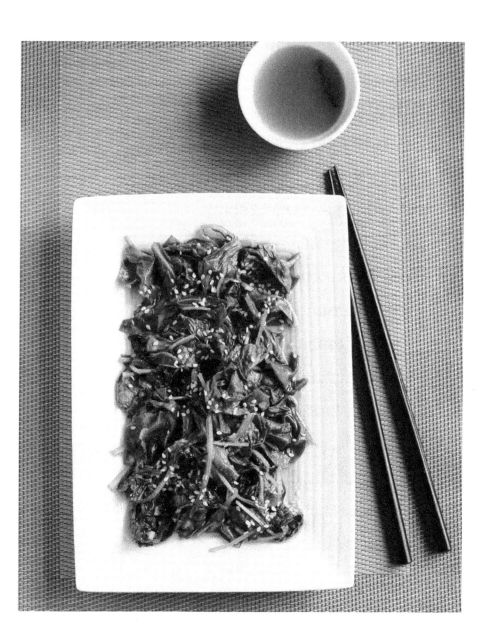

Asparagus Spanakopita

Preparation Time: 25 minutes

Cooking Time: 25 minutes

Servings: 12

Ingredients:

- 2 cups cut fresh asparagus (1-inch pieces)
- 20 sheets phyllo dough, (14 inches x 9 inches)
- Nonstick cooking spray
- Refrigerated butter-flavored spray
- 2 cups torn fresh spinach
- 3 oz. crumbled feta cheese
- 2 tablespoon butter
- 1/4 cup all-purpose flour
- 1-1/2 cups coconut milk
- 3 tablespoon lemon juice
- 1 teaspoon dill weed
- 1 teaspoon dried thyme
- 1/4 teaspoon salt

Directions:

1. In a steamer basket, put the asparagus and place it on top of a saucepan with 1-inch of

water, then boil. Put the cover and let it steam for 5 minutes or until it becomes crisp-tender.

2. Put 1 sheet of phyllo dough in a cooking spray-coated 13x9-inch baking dish, then cut if needed. Use the butter-flavored spray to spritz the dough. Redo the layers 9 times. Lay the asparagus, feta cheese, and spinach on top. Cover it using a sheet of phyllo dough, then spritz it using the butter-flavored spray. Redo the process using the leftover phyllo. Slice it into 12 pieces. Let it bake for 15 minutes at 350 degrees F without cover, or until it turns golden brown.

3. To make the sauce, in a small saucepan, melt the butter. Mix in the flour until it becomes smooth, then slowly add the milk. Stir in salt, thyme, dill, and lemon juice, then boil. Let it cook and stir for 5 minutes until it becomes thick. Serve the spanakopita with the sauce.

Nutrition: Calories 112 Fat 4 Carbs 14 Protein 5

Black Bean and Corn Salsa from Red Gold

Preparation Time: 15 minutes

Cooking Time: 15 minutes

Servings: 25

Ingredients:

- 2 cans black beans, drained and rinsed
- 1 can whole kernel corn, drained
- 2 cans RED GOLD® Petite Diced Tomatoes & Green Chilies
- 1 can RED GOLD® Diced Tomatoes, drained
- 1/2 cup chopped green onions
- 2 tablespoon chopped fresh cilantro
- Salt and black pepper to taste

Directions:

1. Mix all ingredients to combine in a big bowl. Refrigerate to blend flavors for a few hours to overnight. Serve with chips or crackers.

Nutrition: Calories 65 Fat 3 Carbs 8 Protein 9

Avocado Bean Dip

Preparation Time: 15 minutes

Cooking Time: 15 minutes

Servings: 2

Ingredients:

- 1 medium ripe avocado, peeled and cubed
- 1/2 cup fresh cilantro leaves
- 3 tablespoon lime juice
- 1/2 teaspoon onion powder
- 1/2 teaspoon garlic powder
- 1/2 teaspoon chipotle hot pepper sauce
- 1/4 teaspoon salt
- 1/4 teaspoon ground cumin
- Baked tortilla chips

Directions:

1. Mix the first 9 ingredients in a food processor, then cover and blend until smooth. Serve along with chips.

Nutrition: Calories 85 Fat 4 Carbs 13 Protein 6

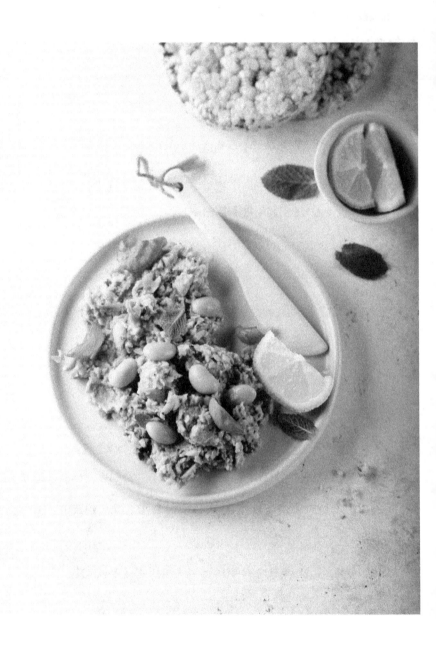

Crunchy Peanut Butter Apple Dip

Preparation Time: 10 minutes

Cooking Time: 10 minutes

Servings: 2

Ingredients:

- 1 carton (8 oz.) reduced-fat spreadable cream cheese
- 1 cup creamy peanut butter
- 1/4 cup coconut milk
- 1 tablespoon brown sugar
- 1 teaspoon vanilla extract
- 1/2 cup chopped unsalted peanuts
- Apple slices

Directions:

1. Beat the initial 5 ingredients in a small bowl until combined. Mix in peanuts. Serve with slices of apple, then put the leftovers in the fridge.

Nutrition: Calories 125 Fat 5 Carbs 23 Protein 9

Creamy Cucumber Yogurt Dip

Preparation Time: 15 minutes

Cooking Time: 15 minutes

Servings: 4

Ingredients:

- 1 cup (8 oz.) reduced-fat plain yogurt
- 4 oz. reduced-fat cream cheese
- 1/2 cup chopped seeded peeled cucumber
- 1-1/2 teaspoon. finely chopped onion
- 1-1/2 teaspoon. snipped fresh dill or 1/2 teaspoon dill weed
- 1 teaspoon lemon juice
- 1 teaspoon grated lemon peel
- 1 garlic clove, minced
- 1/4 teaspoon salt
- 1/4 teaspoon pepper
- Assorted fresh vegetables

Directions:

1. Mix the cream cheese and yogurt in a small bowl. Stir in pepper, salt, garlic, peel, lemon juice, dill, onion, and cucumber. Put on the

cover and let it chill in the fridge. Serve it with the veggies.

Nutrition: Calories 55 Fat 4 Carbs 12 Protein 6

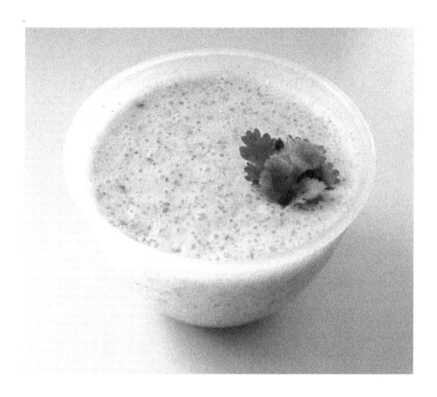

Chunky Cucumber Salsa

Preparation Time: 20 minutes

Cooking Time: 20 minutes

Servings: 4

Ingredients:

- 3 medium cucumbers, peeled and coarsely chopped
- 1 medium mango, coarsely chopped
- 1 cup frozen corn, thawed
- 1 medium sweet red pepper, coarsely chopped
- 1 small red onion, coarsely chopped
- 1 jalapeno pepper, finely chopped
- 3 garlic cloves, minced
- 2 tablespoon white wine vinegar
- 1 tablespoon minced fresh cilantro
- 1 teaspoon salt
- 1/2 teaspoon sugar
- 1/4 to 1/2 teaspoon cayenne pepper

Directions:

1. Mix all ingredients in a big bowl, then chill, covered, about 2 to 3 hours before serving.

Nutrition: Calories 215 Fat 5 Carbs 23 Protein 10

Low-fat Stuffed Mushrooms

Preparation Time: 20 minutes

Cooking Time: 25 minutes

Servings: 6

Ingredients:

- 1 lb. large fresh mushrooms
- 3 tablespoons seasoned bread crumbs
- 3 tablespoons fat-free sour cream
- 2 tablespoons grated Parmesan cheese
- 2 tablespoons minced chives
- 2 tablespoons reduced-fat mayonnaise
- 2 teaspoons balsamic vinegar
- 2 to 3 drops hot pepper sauce, optional

Directions:

1. Take out the stems from the mushrooms, then put the cups aside. Chop the stems and set aside 1/3 cup (get rid of the leftover stems or reserve for later use).
2. Mix the reserved mushroom stems, hot pepper sauce if preferred, vinegar, mayonnaise, chives, Parmesan cheese, sour cream, and breadcrumbs in a bowl, then stir well.

3. Put the mushroom caps on a cooking spray-coated baking tray and stuff it with the crumb mixture.

4. Let it boil for 5 to 7 minutes, placed 4-6 inches from the heat source, or until it turns light brown.

Nutrition: Calories 435 Fat 4 Carbs 23 Protein 9

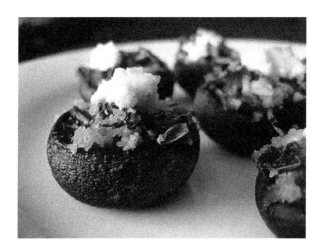

Maple Bagel Spread

Preparation Time: 10 minutes

Cooking Time: 10 minutes

Servings: 1

Ingredients:

- cream cheese
- maple syrup
- cinnamon
- walnuts

Directions:

1. Beat the cinnamon, syrup, and cream cheese in a big bowl until it becomes smooth, then mix in walnuts.

2. Let it chill until ready to serve. Serve it with bagels.

Nutrition: Calories 586 Fat 7 Carbs 23 Protein 4

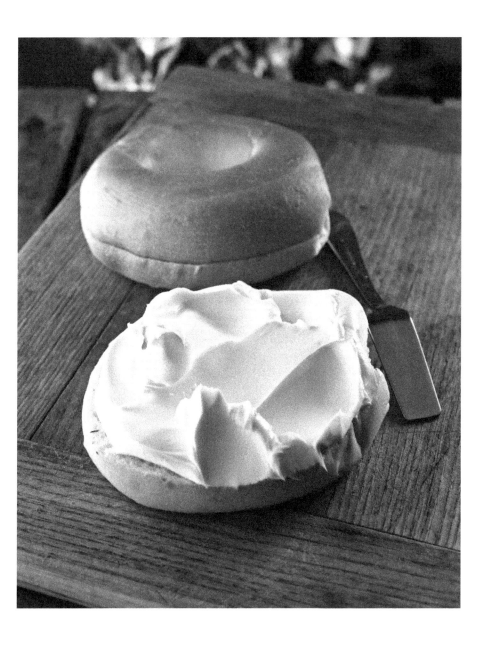

Italian Stuffed Artichokes

Preparation Time: 20 minutes

Cooking Time: 25 minutes

Servings: 4

Ingredients:

- 4 large artichokes
- 2 teaspoon lemon juice
- 2 cups soft Italian bread crumbs, toasted
- 1/2 cup grated Parmigiano-Reggiano cheese
- 1/2 cup minced fresh parsley
- 2 teaspoon Italian seasoning
- 1 teaspoon grated lemon peel
- 1/2 teaspoon pepper
- 1/4 teaspoon salt
- 1 tablespoon olive oil

Directions:

1. Level the bottom of each artichoke using a sharp knife and trim off 1-inch from the tops. Snip off tips of outer leaves using kitchen scissors, then brush lemon juice on cut edges. In a Dutch oven, stand the artichokes and pour

1-inch of water, then boil. Lower the heat, put the cover, and let it simmer for 5 minutes or until the leaves near the middle pull out effortlessly.

2. Turn the artichokes upside down to drain. Allow it to stand for 10 minutes. Carefully scrape out the fuzzy middle part of the artichokes using a spoon and get rid of it.

3. Mix the salt, pepper, lemon peel, Italian seasoning, garlic, parsley, cheese, and breadcrumbs in a small bowl, then add olive oil and stir well. Gently spread the artichoke leaves apart, then fill it with breadcrumb mixture.

4. Put it in a cooking spray-coated 11x7-inch baking dish. Let it bake for 10 minutes at 350 degrees F without cover, or until the filling turns light brown.

Nutrition: Calories 543 Fat 5 Carbs 44 Protein 6

Enchilada sauce

Preparation Time: 10 minutes

Cooking Time: 10 minutes

Servings: 13

Ingredients:

- 1½ tablespoon MCT oil
- ½ tablespoon chili powder
- ½ tablespoon whole wheat flour
- ½ teaspoon ground cumin
- ¼ teaspoon oregano (dried or fresh)
- ¼ teaspoon salt (or to taste)
- 1 garlic clove (minced)
- 1 tablespoon tomato paste
- 1 cup vegetable broth
- ½ teaspoon apple vinegar
- ½ teaspoon ground black pepper

Directions:

1. Heat a small saucepan over medium heat.
2. Add the MCT oil and minced garlic to the pan and sauté for about 1 minute.
3. Mix the dry spices and flour in a medium bowl and pour the dry mixture into the saucepan.

4. Stir in the tomato paste immediately, and slowly pour in the vegetable broth, making sure that everything combines well.

5. When everything is mixed thoroughly, bring up the heat to medium-high until it gets to a simmer and cook for about 3 minutes or until the sauce becomes a bit thicker.

6. Remove the pan from the heat and add the vinegar with the black pepper, adding more salt and pepper to taste.

Nutrition: Calories 225 Fat 4 Carbs 33 Protein 5

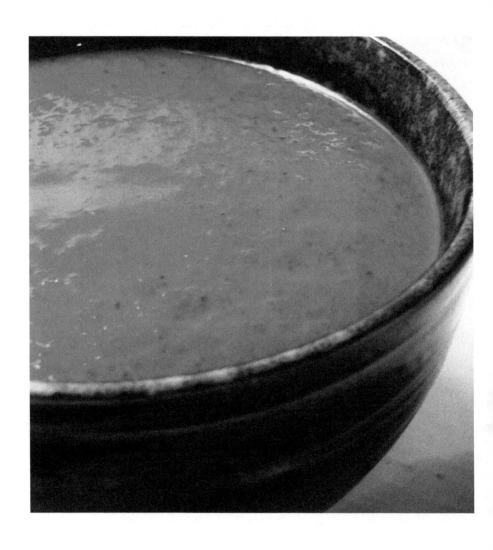

Stir Fry Noodles

Preparation Time: 10 minutes

Cooking Time: 8 minutes

Servings: 4

Ingredients:

- 1 cup broccoli, chopped
- 1 cup red bell pepper, chopped
- 1 cup mushrooms, chopped
- 1 large onion, chopped
- 1 batch Stir Fry Sauce, prepared
- Salt and black pepper, to taste
- 2 cups spaghetti, cooked
- 4 garlic cloves, minced
- 2 tablespoons sesame oil

Directions:

1. Heat sesame oil in a pan over medium heat and add garlic, onions, bell pepper, broccoli, mushrooms.
2. Sauté for about 5 minutes and add spaghetti noodles and stir fry sauce.
3. Mix well and cook for 3 more minutes.
4. Dish out in plates and serve to enjoy.

Nutrition: Calories: 567 Total fat: 48g Total carbs: 6g Fiber: 4g; Net carbs: 2g Sodium: 373mg Protein: 33g

Spicy Sweet Chili Veggie Noodles

Preparation Time: 10 minutes

Cooking Time: 7 minutes

Servings: 2

Ingredients:

- 1 head of broccoli, cut into bite sized florets
- 1 onion, finely sliced
- 1 tablespoon olive oil
- 1 courgette, halved
- 2 nests of whole-wheat noodles
- 150g mushrooms, sliced
- For Sauce
- 3 tablespoons soy sauce
- ¼ cup sweet chili sauce
- 1 teaspoon Sriracha
- 1 tablespoon peanut butter
- 2 tablespoons boiled water
- For Topping
- 2 teaspoons sesame seeds
- 2 teaspoons dried chili flakes

Directions:

1. Heat olive oil on medium heat in a saucepan and add onions.
2. Sauté for about 2 minutes and add broccoli, courgette and mushrooms.
3. Cook for about 5 minutes, stirring occasionally.
4. Whisk sweet chili sauce, soy sauce, Sriracha, water and peanut butter in a bowl.
5. Cook the noodles according to packet instructions and add to the vegetables.
6. Stir in the sauce and top with dried chili flakes and sesame seeds to serve.

Nutrition: Calories: 351 Total Fat: 27g Protein: 25g Total Carbs: 2g Fiber: 1g Net Carbs: 1g

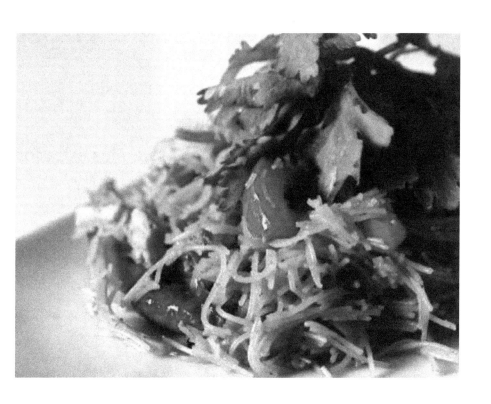

Creamy Vegan Mushroom Pasta

Preparation Time: 10 minutes

Cooking Time: 30 minutes

Servings: 6

Ingredients:

- 2 cups frozen peas, thawed
- 3 tablespoons flour, unbleached
- 3 cups almond breeze, unsweetened
- 1 tablespoon nutritional yeast
- 1/3 cup fresh parsley, chopped, plus extra for garnish
- ¼ cup olive oil
- 1 pound pasta of choice
- 4 cloves garlic, minced
- 2/3 cup shallots, chopped
- 8 cups mixed mushrooms, sliced
- Salt and black pepper, to taste

Directions:

1. Take a bowl and boil pasta in salted water.
2. Heat olive oil in a pan over medium heat.
3. Add mushrooms, garlic, shallots and ½ tsp salt and cook for 15 minutes.

4. Sprinkle flour on the vegetables and stir for a minute while cooking.
5. Add almond beverage, stir constantly.
6. Let it simmer for 5 minutes and add pepper to it.
7. Cook for 3 more minutes and remove from heat.
8. Stir in nutritional yeast.
9. Add peas, salt, and pepper.
10. Cook for another minute and add
11. Add pasta to this sauce.
12. Garnish and serve!

Nutrition: Calories: 364 Total Fat: 28g Protein: 24g Total Carbs: 4g Fiber: 2g Net Carbs: 2g

Vegetable Penne Pasta

Preparation Time: 15 minutes

Cooking Time: 20 minutes

Servings: 6

Ingredients:

- ½ large onion, chopped
- 2 celery sticks, chopped
- ½ tablespoon ginger paste
- ½ cup green bell pepper
- 1½ tablespoons soy sauce
- ½ teaspoon parsley
- Salt and black pepper, to taste
- ½ pound penne pasta, cooked
- 2 large carrots, diced
- ½ small leek, chopped
- 1 tablespoon olive oil
- ½ teaspoon garlic paste
- ½ tablespoon Worcester sauce
- ½ teaspoon coriander
- 1 cup water

Directions:

1. Heat olive oil in a wok on medium heat and add onions, garlic and ginger paste.
2. Sauté for about 3 minutes and stir in all bell pepper, celery sticks, carrots and leek.
3. Sauté for about 5 minutes and add remaining ingredients except for pasta.
4. Cover the lid and cook for about 12 minutes.
5. Stir in the cooked pasta and dish out to serve warm.

Nutrition: Calories: 385 Total Fat: 29g Protein: 26g Total Carbs: 5g Fiber: 1g Net Carbs: 4g

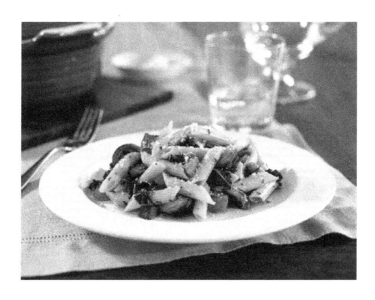

Creamy Vegan Spinach Pasta

Preparation Time: 20 minutes

Cooking Time: 5 minutes

Servings: 4

Ingredients:

- 1 cup raw cashews, soaked in water for 8 hours
- 2 tablespoons lemon juice
- 1 tablespoon olive oil
- 1½ cups vegetable broth
- 2 tablespoons fresh dill, chopped
- Red pepper flakes, to taste
- 10 ounces dried fusilli
- ½ cup almond milk, unflavored and unsweetened
- 2 tablespoons white miso paste
- 4 garlic cloves, divided
- 8-ounces fresh spinach, finely chopped
- ¼ cup scallions, chopped
- Salt and black pepper, to taste

Directions:

1. Boil salted water in a large pot and add pasta.

2. Cook according to the package directions and drain the pasta into a colander.

3. Dish out the pasta in a large serving bowl and add a dash of olive oil to prevent sticking.

4. Put the cashews, milk, miso, lemon juice, and 1 garlic clove into the food processor and blend until smooth.

5. Put olive oil over medium heat in a large pot and add the remaining 3 cloves of garlic.

6. Sauté for about 1 minute and stir in the spinach and broth.

7. Raise the heat and allow to simmer for about 4 minutes until the spinach is bright green and wilted.

8. Stir in the pasta and cashew mixture and season with salt and black pepper.

9. Top with scallions and dill and dish out into plates to serve.

Nutrition: Calories: 94 Total Fat: 10g Protein: 0g Total Carbs: 1g Fiber: 0.3g Net Carbs: 0.7g